WHY F[barcode C000121408]
FAIL AT FITNESS

The *10 Major Mistakes*
People Unwittingly Make Causing Them to be Unfit, Stressed, Tired, Overweight and Suffering Aches & Pains

Oct 2018,
My dear friend Caroline.
Enjoy your Healthy Fitness!
Kerrison.

By Kerrison Preston BSc Hons Biochem, BSc Ost, DipPT, MTCUGB
Osteopath, Fitness Consultant,
Advanced Tai Chi Instructor

- Helped more than 7,800 individuals, including Olympic gold and silver medalists and stars of stage and screen
- Ten years advisor to an elite military extreme sports team
- University lecturer in Anatomy and Clinical Studies

- Creator of 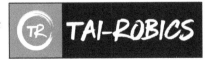 TAI-ROBICS

Publishing in the United Kingdom by:
Kerrison Preston

Book design & layout by Velin@Perseus-Design.com

ISBN Number: 978-1-64440-577-2 (Paperback)

Big, big thanks to everyone at Peter Thomson International for their advice, guidance, support and patience. I could not have created Tai-Robics or produced this book without their help.
www.peterthomson.com

About the author

As an Honours graduate in Biochemistry, Kerrison went straight into Public Relations and Marketing in the biotechnology industry then moved into business software - putting him through all the ups and downs of the corporate workplace. By age 26 he was UK Public Relations Manager at what was then the world's largest PC business software company.

He started learning Tai Chi (Chinese yoga/kung fu) in 1986, which got him thinking about health. So he did four years hard studying for his degree in Osteopathy, graduating aged 31 with a baby and a toddler and total assets of £200.

He founded his own clinic in 1994, which he built up into a leading regional natural health centre. He also qualified as a Fitness Consultant and studied nutritional health management.

In 2001 he became an advisor to the Red Devils Freefall Team, the display team of the British Army Parachute Regiment, who trained him in skydiving. In 2008 he joined the first ever expedition to skydive at Mount Everest - giving him a full minute of freefall above the Himalayas.

Kerrison taught Anatomy, Osteopathic Technique and Clinical Studies at Oxford Brookes University.

Tai-Robics, Kerrison's unique exercise system, emerged by combining the best of Tai Chi and yoga with the best of Western sports science. He created Tai-Robics to fill the gaps left wide open by other exercise systems.

You are a living, breathing, active human being.

You have hopes and fears, wins and losses, ups and downs.

You're doing your best to cope with the demands of life.

Just like me.

You've probably wanted to be fit and healthy.

Perhaps you hoped for the energy, happiness and power to charge forwards into achievement and success.

But life got in the way.

Aches, pains, stress, tiredness and a bulging waistline crept in and dragged you down.

Just like me.

And just like millions of others too.

I've seen it again and again with my patients and clients.

It was getting me too.

It took me years to work out what was wrong.

My training had made me think I was doing the right thing. I was doing what the experts told me, what the science and research said was best.

And yet…. it wasn't really working, for me and for millions of others.

My clothes were getting tighter. My energy was wilting. All around me the "obesity crisis" was getting worse and healthcare round the world was creaking with the strain.

Without even knowing it, I, along with everyone else, was making ten Major Mistakes.

Perhaps it's been the same for you.

Just like me.

Ten Major Mistakes.

And here they are.........

The Ten Major Mistakes That Can Make You Unwittingly Fail At Fitness

1 Fitness = Health....? 9

2 Out Of Your Head & Out Of Your Body 15

3 Busting The Thermostat...21

4 Gasping For Air...27

5 Going In Cold..33

6 Shock - Horror..39

7 Stiff As a Board 45

8 High As a Damaged Kite..51

9 Rubbish In, Rubbish Out 57

10 Too Much, Too Soon...65

Notes and thoughts:

1
Fitness = Health.....?

Which do you want? Fitness or Health? Well, obviously, ideally you want both! And they're the same thing, anyway…. aren't they?

Surely getting fit makes you healthy,… doesn't it?

That's exactly what stops you getting either.

Have you noticed how sport is everywhere?

Hot, sweaty sport. Olympics. Tennis. Football. Rugby. Cycling. Huge crowds of marathon runners. The list is endless.

Inspiring?

Motivating?

Or disheartening?

It's just so much effort! You know you should. It's meant to be so good for you. But then you possibly know some super-fit people who constantly get colds and injuries.

And it's such a hassle. Finding the time. Getting to the gym. Washing the sweat off your body and out of your hair. Then you can hardly move the next day anyway.

The thing is, probably no-one's ever told you there's a world of difference between exercising for "fitness" and exercising for "health".

Fitness is good. Fitness is great. It gets you ready for that big event. It helps you enjoy your other sports.

It can also knock you sideways!

It stresses you and pushes you to extremes. That's fine for a while but you can't "peak" forever.

And that's the very heart of the problem.

Think about it…

Sport is a multi-trillion-dollar global industry. Top stars are paid fortunes. Governments spend billions on building enormous stadia and organising huge international events. Vast sums are invested in finding and training the best athletes.

Follow the money and you find the research focuses on getting top athletes up to their peak performance - and keeping them there for as long as their bodies hold out.

They focus on "fitness" while "health" is thrown out the window.

Focusing on fitness sets you up to fail.

Long-term fitness training damages your health.

Why do you think there are so few sports professionals who manage to carry on into their 30s? Let alone their 40s!? Roger Federer and the Williams sisters are amongst the extremely rare exceptions that prove a general rule.

A successful sports career follows a notoriously brutal pathway. Only a very small percentage make it through to the top. Thousands of would-be athletes fall by the wayside then suffer the long-term after-effects of their years of training.

I've seen this particularly with my military and ex-military patients. Being fit for the battlefield in your 20s doesn't do you any good when you're in your 50s!

Almost all commercial exercise programmes are based on the methods designed for keeping young top athletes at peak fitness. They use intense and potentially dangerous activities. You have to be healthy enough to cope with the damage they can cause you.

Of particular concern is a condition called rhabdomyolysis in which over-worked muscles fall apart and release kidney-damaging toxins. There have been more and more cases of people ending up in hospital following exercise classes, sometimes rushed straight from the gym.

As such, those programmes are simply not appropriate for the vast majority of people. They're not even really appropriate for athletes! Think what you could achieve with an athlete's constitution if you exercised for health rather than burning yourself out in your 30s.

People do give it a go. They try. They buy the equipment. They buy the books and DVDs and online programmes. They join the gym. Some of them are healthy enough to succeed, despite the damage.

But I bet you know at least one person who has given up and Failed at Fitness.

Perhaps that person was you?

Health does not follow fitness. You have to be healthy enough to get fit in the first place. It is far better to focus on exercising to become healthy rather than fit. It is absolutely essential to get healthy first - then you can get fit.

Focus on health instead and fitness follows naturally. You gain agility, energy, confidence, happiness and long-term achievement, right the way through into old age. You're also ready and primed for when you want peak fitness as well.

Thinking Fitness is the same as Health makes you:

- Exercise the wrong way;
- Push yourself to dangerous extremes;
- Risk lasting injuries;
- Risk burning out and giving up;
- Do yourself long-term damage;
- Pay for it in later life!

So the first Major Mistake is: **Thinking Fitness Equals Health.**

The solution: Understand the difference between exercising for Health and exercising for Fitness - carry on reading this book! Then focus your exercise programme on health rather than fitness. Become healthy enough to get fit, properly fit - fit for life as well as for sport. Boost your health and you'll find fitness follows naturally.

Your best and healthiest exercise programme:

1   Focuses on health first, fitness second

2   ?

3   ?

4   ?

5   ?

6   ?

7   ?

8   ?

9   ?

10   ?

2
Out Of Your Head &
Out Of Your Body

Empty stomach. Full bladder or bowels. Pain.

That's it. That's your "Inside World".

Everything else comes from your "Outside World".

That's why it's hard to be healthy.

Try this, right now:

Put your left hand out in front of you, fingers out straight, thumb at the top, little finger at the bottom. Point at the centre of your left palm with the tip of your right index finger, with about an inch between them. Or point at your foot instead, if necessary.

Move your left hand around while keeping the tip of your right finger the same distance away at all times.

Easy, yes?

Now do it with your eyes shut. You can't see what's happening. But you should still be able to do it.

Still easy, yes?

You've just experienced your sixth sense. Your real sixth sense. It's nothing to do with seeing ghosts! It's all about your sense of physical self awareness.

There are five senses for your outside world: Sight, hearing, smell, taste and touch.

Your sixth sense, proprioception (pro-pree-oh-sep-shun), deals with your inside world. It tells you the position of your joints, the tightness of your muscles, the stretching of your skin. It tells you how you stand, sit and move.

Just now, your brain was receiving information from your left arm and sending instructions to your right arm - without you even thinking about it.

You see, the conscious mind largely ignores proprioception. The other five senses, especially vision, barge it out the way. People overwhelmingly focus on the outside world - except for hunger, fullness and pain.

They lose awareness of their physical self. Then they sit, stand, move and breathe badly. So they end up tired, stressed and aching, perhaps with shoulders pulled up to their ears and a pounding headache.

Does that sound familiar?

I notice it all the time with my patients and clients. "Just relax your arm" I say. "It is relaxed" they insist, while holding it up in the air. They're always amazed when they start becoming aware of the difference between relaxed and working muscle - feeling that difference from the inside.

Hardly any sports positively encourage you to be properly tuned in to your proprioception. If they do at all, they tend to emphasise only the safety aspects of good form - such as guarding your lower back when weight-lifting - rather than actively helping you become more aware of yourself.

It makes a significant difference. By exercising in a way that actively encourages your conscious proprioception - being aware of your joints and muscles, your posture, your balance, your breathing, your co-ordination - you will gain much better quality of movement. Not only will you have more energy and fewer aches and pains in every day life, you will also leap up a level in your performance in other sports.

Tuning in to your proprioception, your sense of physical and postural self-awareness, is an essential part of the process of exercising for better health, letting fitness follow naturally.

Losing conscious awareness of your proprioception makes you:

- Have poorer quality movement;
- Sit, stand, move and breathe badly;
- Prone to unconscious muscular tension;
- Have aches, pains and stress;
- Tire more easily;
- Not reach your full potential in sport.

So the second Major Mistake is: **Lack of Physical Self-Awareness.**

The solution: Rediscover your physical self with exercise specially designed to bring your proprioception back into conscious awareness. You'll be amazed at the difference, whatever your current level of health and fitness. You'll gain better posture, movement and co-ordination. You'll have more energy and fewer aches and pains. Your other sports will leap up a level.

Your best and healthiest exercise programme:

1   Focuses on health first, fitness second

2   Boosts your physical self-awareness

3   ?

4   ?

5   ?

6   ?

7   ?

8   ?

9   ?

10   ?

Notes and thoughts:

3
Busting The Thermostat

Your biochemistry works best at about 37°C.

Getting too hot messes it up.

Your brain absolutely cannot cope with overheating. A 4°C increase in brain temperature can kill you.

So getting rid of excessive heat takes priority over everything:

- Supplying oxygen, nutrients, water and fuel;
- Clearing away toxins.

Everything.

Everything is pushed down the priority list.

Getting rid of that dangerous heat becomes an urgent emergency.

That's why you sweat. Sweat cools you down by evaporating from your skin and taking heat with it.

Hard-exercising muscles create amazing amounts of heat. They also need lots of blood to bring in oxygen, nutrients, water and fuel - and to take away toxic biochemical waste.

That same blood carries the heat away too, taking it to the skin for sweat to get rid of.

And remember, getting rid of the heat is the number one priority.

Blood should be picking up oxygen from the lungs plus nutrients and fuel from the liver and gut, carrying them to the muscles, heart and brain then going back for more. It should also be taking away toxins and getting rid of them through the kidneys.

But it starts focusing on that deadly heat - shuttling between muscles and skin.

So overheating diverts vital blood away from everywhere and into your skin instead.

Your skin is huge. As a whole it is bigger than any other part of your body. It can hold a vast amount of blood - taken away from where it is really needed.

Just when your hard-working muscles are needing maximum blood for nutrition and cleansing it is being shunted off into your skin to get rid of heat!

Go past the temperature tipping point with exercise and you starve your muscles, heart and brain just when they're most hungry.

The paradox of hot and sweaty exercise!

Changing sweat from liquid to vapour is the key part of the cooling process. Liquid water molecules like to stay close together. It takes a lot of heat to make them spread out and evaporate into the air.

But there's a limit to how well the system works.

Overdo it and you sweat so much that it just drips off you instead of evaporating. If it's dripping rather than evaporating it's not taking away anything like as much heat.

So lots of heat gets left behind.

Then your temperature control system overloads and breaks down.

More and more sweat pours out and more and more blood floods into your skin, sometimes even making you go bright red. And you go on sweating even when you've stopped exercising.

Your body is desperately trying to get rid of that deadly heat.

But it's using a system that has stopped working!

Is it any wonder that organisers of sports events have to be prepared for people collapsing from heat exhaustion?

If someone is bright red with sweat pouring off them then you know they're in trouble.

One last point...

You probably already know that sweat is salty. It also contains many other important minerals and vitamins, which would normally be helping your biochemistry work properly. You lose them when you sweat excessively.

If you're dripping sweat, you're overdoing it. If you get hot and sweaty every time you exercise, you're doing yourself more harm than good.

You are far better off exercising to get warm but not overheated, so your blood goes where it's needed. Then your brain, heart, muscles and other organs get the oxygen and nutrients they need and their biochemical waste toxins are cleared away.

This brings us back, again, to the first Major Mistake. Exercising within your natural range of temperature control is an important part of the process of becoming healthy enough to get fit.

Hot and sweaty exercise:

- Messes up your biochemistry;
- Stresses your brain;
- Overloads your temperature control system;
- Diverts blood away from where it is most needed;
- Reduces fuel and oxygen for your muscles, heart and brain;
- Builds up toxic biochemical waste;
- Dehydrates you;
- Wastes minerals and vitamins.

So the third Major Mistake is: **Getting Hot and Sweaty.**

The solution: Build your health and fitness on a core foundation of exercise that warms you but doesn't overheat you - have sweat evaporating rather than dripping. So you minimise dehydration and your blood goes where it's needed, nourishing and cleansing your tissues and leaving you feeling refreshed and energised.

Your best and healthiest exercise:

1   Focuses on health first, fitness second

2   Boosts your physical self-awareness

3   Keeps you at a safe temperature

4   ?

5   ?

6   ?

7   ?

8   ?

9   ?

10   ?

4

Gasping For Air

Glucose, from your food, is your main fuel, particularly in your brain.

Your brain uses a vast percentage of the glucose floating in your bloodstream. It also uses about a fifth of the oxygen. Given its size, this is way out of proportion relative to the rest of your body.

Your muscles and heart use lots of glucose too, especially when you're exercising.

With oxygen, glucose gives you loads of energy.

Without oxygen, glucose gives you only a tiny bit of energy. And produces lots of toxins.

You can get even more energy out of fat. But you can't use fat as fuel at all without oxygen. Run out of oxygen and your fat-burning just stops dead.

So if you're not getting enough oxygen you stop burning fat and your muscles and heart accumulate toxins. They can get really painful, eventually just giving up and stopping.

Energy is extracted by chopping up the fuel molecules, which releases carbon atoms. If there's no oxygen, the carbon atoms are made into toxins. Oxygen helps extract far more energy and carries away the carbon atoms by forming carbon dioxide. Your body detects the increasing carbon dioxide. That's what makes you pant.

If you're panting, it means too much oxygen has been used up. Your lungs desperately try to get more oxygen and get rid of the carbon dioxide. Your heart goes into overdrive trying to pump oxygen to your muscles, to itself and to your brain.

Just like with overheating, your brain really doesn't like getting low on oxygen. Remember, your brain needs far more glucose, plus the oxygen necessary for safely and efficiently extracting the energy, than any other part of your body. Unless your brain is very cold, which it won't be when you're exercising, five minutes without oxygen is enough to turn it off completely and permanently - serious damage if not actual death.

You carry on panting even when you've stopped exercising. That's to pay off the "oxygen debt", your oxygen overdraft. You have to get back up to normal levels <u>and</u> pay interest with extra oxygen needed for getting rid of the toxins.

The glucose floating freely in your muscles and blood is the first fuel to be used when you start exercising. After a while you start releasing the extra glucose stored in your muscles and liver.

If you carry on exercising your body starts to activate its stores of fat as well.

Remember, fat contains far more energy than glucose. Fat is an excellent fuel. As long as there's plenty of oxygen available.

Your body's first question when switching to fat-burning is "Is there plenty of oxygen?"

If the answer is "Yes" then it burns more and more fat.

Possibly exactly what you want and need!

But if the answer is "No" your body does precisely the opposite.

If there isn't enough oxygen your body leaves your fat where it is and goes back to burning glucose.

And doing it very inefficiently.

And producing lots of toxins.

What's more, if you're gasping for breath when exercising there's a good chance you're dripping sweat too! So not only have you started running out of oxygen but you've also overheated and diverted a huge amount of blood into your skin, making it even harder to get oxygen to where it's needed.

Double trouble!

And that's not all of it either. There's more:

You breathe best when you use your diaphragm, the dome-shaped muscle underneath your lungs. It stretches your lungs downwards, pushing your tummy out as it does so, which also helps keep your digestive system mobile and healthy. You should only ever need to use your ribs or shoulders for breathing when you have to pay off the oxygen debt created by over-exercising.

Poor proprioception and poor posture stop you using your diaphragm properly, so you get out of breath even more quickly. Using your ribs and/or shoulders for breathing when you're not doing hard exercise is a sure sign that something is wrong.

Are you starting to see how these Major Mistakes connect to each other?

Repeatedly getting very out of breath does you more harm than good. So does repeatedly overheating. They are both also affected by your sense of physical self-awareness, or lack of it - posture, movement, awareness of your muscles and joints.

And they are vital parts in the process of exercising for "Health" rather than "Fitness".

Vast numbers of people regularly force themselves into getting hot and sweaty and out of breath, thinking they are getting "fit". They're not. They're hurting themselves. Then, guess what, they give up and they Fail at Fitness!

You have to be healthy enough to get fit.

Get healthy first.

Then get fit.

Panting and gasping for breath:

- Means you're running out of oxygen;
- Stops you using fat as fuel;
- Makes you use glucose very inefficiently;
- Builds up toxins;
- Stresses your brain, heart, muscles and other organs.

So the fourth Major Mistake is: **Getting Out of Breath.**

The solution: Build your health and fitness on a core foundation of exercise that is specially designed to get you breathing properly again and keeping you fully oxygenated while you exercise, so you get more energy from your food, burn fat and avoid building up toxins.

Your best and healthiest exercise programme:

1   Focuses on health first, fitness second

2   Boosts your physical self-awareness

3   Keeps you at a safe temperature

4   Gives you all the oxygen you need

5   ?

6   ?

7   ?

8   ?

9   ?

10   ?

5
Going In Cold

Going straight into vigorous exercise without warming up puts you at risk of injury.

Have you noticed how it can take a few seconds to get moving again if you've been sitting still for a long time?

Perhaps it's after a long car journey or hours at your desk or watching a film. You might need to give your legs and arms a bit of a shake to get the blood flowing and the muscles working.

You are changing state, going from staying still to moving around. It can take a little while for your body to catch up with what your mind wants it to do.

The same principle applies when you start exercising.

You are going from a state of gentle movement to one of vigorous movement.

It takes a bit of time for your body to catch up - for your blood vessels to open, for your muscles to be able to work faster and harder, for your lungs to breathe deeper, for your heart to pump harder.

Making your muscles work hard when they're not ready can use up their available oxygen very quickly (they usually have just enough for emergencies - in case a lion suddenly jumps out at you). So they rapidly go into the inefficient and toxin-producing way of using glucose.

You've now got toxins in your muscles - while you're still expecting them to work hard. You face the risk of cramps, strains and tears. Even if you avoid real injury you are still highly likely to be sore the next day.

Have you ever been sore the day after exercising?

Now, you may well be thinking "Yeah, but everyone knows you have to warm up. And I do warm up. Every time."

That's great. I'm very pleased to hear it.

It also brings me to the key point of this particular Major Mistake…

The "warm-up", if it happens at all, is often far too vigorous and intense in itself!

I've seen it again and again with so many of my patients and clients, even top athletes. I've lost count of the number of people I have had to help discover how to warm up properly.

A prime example was a top competitive martial artist. He kept getting injuries until I made him increase his pre-bout warm-up from five minutes to half an hour. Yes, half an hour - six times as long.

I remember it myself from when I was on the receiving end - energetically running up and down the rugby field or back and forth across the dojo for a few minutes before doing the "real" exercise.

Substituting one form of vigorous exercise for another is not a proper warm up! You're still going straight in from cold.

It needs to be done gradually. Very gradually. That's the whole point of warming up!

Wake your body up slowly, bit by bit. Give it a chance to keep up with what your mind is demanding of it. Give it time to get the blood flowing, to get the nutrients and oxygen to where they're needed. Give it time to start burning fat.

Give yourself time to activate.

If you're already regularly doing any sport I suggest you double or triple your warm-up time at the very least, possibly even more.

And start much more gently than you have been.

You'll be amazed at the difference it makes. You'll have more energy and stamina. You'll have fewer aches and pains and fewer injuries.

Or, perhaps, use an exercise programme that has a proper warm-up built into it…

Not warming up properly:

- Risks repeated and lasting injury;
- Reduces your fat-burning;
- Builds up toxins;
- Overloads your biochemistry;
- Reduces the benefits of your workout;
- Stops you performing at your best;

So the fifth Major Mistake is: **Not Warming Up Properly**.

The solution: Double or triple your warm-up time, or even more. Warm up very gradually, slowly increasing the intensity bit by bit.

Or use an exercise programme that naturally includes a proper, safe warm-up.

Your best and healthiest exercise programme:

1   Focuses on health first, fitness second

2   Boosts your physical self-awareness

3   Keeps you at a safe temperature

4   Gives you all the oxygen you need

5   Activates you gradually and safely

6   ?

7   ?

8   ?

9   ?

10   ?

Notes and thoughts:

6
Shock - Horror

Repeated shock impacts and sudden strains damage your bones, joints, ligaments and muscles. Your shins, knees and the base of your back are particularly at risk.

Like all life, from bacteria to blue whales, you are made of cells. A cell is basically a tiny closed-off bag of water. Floating inside is a mix of molecular structures for doing the cell's biochemistry - getting energy from food plus anything specific for particular tissues.

Some parts of you are made almost entirely of cells - billions of them - e.g. your brain or liver.

Other parts, such as your bones, have relatively few cells. Instead, they're made of stuff produced by the cells. Different cells produce different stuff for different tissues.

The cells in bone constantly dissolve it and rebuild it. They do this along the lines of force. So bones are strongest where most needed.

This works really well with forces that are applied and increased gradually - giving the cells clear instructions for strengthening the bone.

Sudden forces can have the opposite effect.

The force of a shock impact can crack any weak spots, which then have to be repaired.

And that's the problem.

Repaired bone isn't as good as bone that's been properly maintained.

Repaired bone is laid down quickly, any old how. It then takes a while for the cells to make it strong again.

In the meantime, guess what happens if you carry on doing whatever caused the cracks in the first place!

Yup, that's right. You end up with ever more cracks that never get fully repaired. So your bones weaken, risking a much bigger fracture.

"Shin Splints" from running on hard surfaces is a good example - cracks that can make it too painful even just to stand, let alone walk or run.

I've had them. They hurt! Ouch!

You wouldn't be able to move if your skeleton was all one bone. Your joints, where two or more separate bones meet, let you be mobile.

The cartilage that lines your main joints is tough, springy and very slippery. It lets bones slide against each other smoothly and easily. Like bone, it has cells in it to look after it.

But it doesn't get any blood, which only gets as far as the lining around the joint. Nutrients and oxygen drift through the joint's lubricating fluid to get to the cells. The cells' toxic waste does the same in reverse.

Regular, gentle on-off compression squeezes and releases the cartilage like a sponge, getting nutrients in and flushing toxins out - nourishing and cleansing the cells, keeping them alive and healthy.

Repeated shock impacts, however, can make it crack and crumble faster than the cells can repair it - stressing the cells and putting them at risk.

And giving you early arthritis.

If the cells die off, the cartilage can never be repaired at all. It wears away completely and you end up with bone grating directly on bone.

Giving you really bad arthritis - constant back pain or knees and hips that need replacing.

It's the same with the ligaments that hold your joints together and the tendons linking muscle to bone - but with traction rather than compression. Gentle loading tells the cells where to strengthen them. Sudden forces cause tears that might never heal properly.

Lastly, your muscles themselves can be injured by sudden strains too.

A muscle is mainly made of cells - unlike bone. It works by using a molecular ratchet to shorten its cells. This pulls two bones towards each other, which makes a joint move.

Work it or stretch it too hard and too suddenly and it tears. This can be anything from a disruption of the molecular ratchet right the way up to a major rip.

Micro-injuries can stimulate a muscle to grow - as long as it's given enough time and nutrients to repair and recover properly.

41

It's when it doesn't repair properly that you get the problems, whether the injury is large or small. A big muscle full of scar tissue won't be stronger than a healthy small muscle. Scar tissue stops it working properly and risks further injury and permanent pain.

Whether it's bone, cartilage, ligament, tendon or muscle, the key point is that repeatedly injuring it faster than the cells can repair it obviously does more harm than good. Shock impacts and sudden strains are major causes of such injuries.

Remember those top athletes who burn out in their 30s?

Guess what they suffer from in their 40s and 50s!

Do you really want to exercise the same way as them?

Shock impacts and sudden strains:

- Injure your bones, joints and muscles;
- Weaken your bones, cartilage, ligaments, tendons and muscles;
- Can stop you exercising completely;
- Cause permanent tissue damage;
- Overload your repair systems;
- Give you constant pain;
- Make you pay in later life.

So the sixth Major Mistake is: **Exercising with Shock Impacts and Sudden Strains.**

The solution: Exercise in such a way that your bones, joints, ligaments, tendons and muscles are gently and firmly stressed without any shock impacts or sudden strains, so they are strengthened rather than injured.

Your best and healthiest exercise programme:

1   Focuses on health first, fitness second

2   Boosts your physical self-awareness

3   Keeps you at a safe temperature

4   Gives you all the oxygen you need

5   Activates you gradually and safely

6   Safely strengthens you

7   ?

8   ?

9   ?

10   ?

7

Stiff As a Board

Strength, stamina and suppleness are the three pillars of healthy fitness.

Have you noticed what most people do in the gym?

Remember that short and ineffective warm-up they might not even do?

That's when they might do a little bit of stretching.

But they want to get on with the real business of working out with weights or running on the machine - focusing on strength and stamina, the "important" stuff.

The thing is, suppleness underlies the other two. Suppleness is an important part of avoiding the second Major Mistake - lack of physical self awareness - which, along with the first Major Mistake, underlies all the others.

Suppleness helps your whole body work better. It helps you move better, stand better, breathe better. Suppleness massively cuts your risk of injury. It lets you do your strength and stamina work much more safely and effectively.

Your body is a flexible three-dimensional structure that moves around in a gravity field, balanced on one end. It contains natural focal points of mechanical strain. These are the places, like the base of your back, that can give way when overloaded.

Stiffness makes this worse by making you break rather than bend. It creeps up on you as the years go by - muscles tightening, ligaments shortening and thickening. Then you exercise too hard and end up injured. Any further challenge and you can crack like concrete rather than bend and bounce like rubber. So you give up exercising and you Fail at Fitness.

Suppleness, helped by good proprioception, lets you move properly and safely. Mechanical force is spread throughout your body. The force goes where it should and nothing gets overloaded.

The problem comes from the simple fact that very few people really know how to stretch safely and effectively.

One of the key incidents that inspired this book was when I witnessed an experienced instructor getting it completely wrong. This instructor was highly qualified in a well known and popular exercise system that emphasises suppleness. The class was being told to stretch a particularly important muscle. The technique they were obediently applying did precisely the opposite - it very accurately shortened the muscle instead!

The instructor didn't know the anatomy or understand the biomechanics of what the people in the class were being told to do.

I was shocked. It forced me to think about my own knowledge and understanding.

If instructors don't know, how can they teach their clients?

It's no wonder so many people are unwittingly making these Major Mistakes!

Here are the Golden Guidelines for safe and effective stretching:

- Little and Often;
- Gentle and Accurate;
- Allow it to loosen rather than force it to stretch;
- Have some knowledge of the anatomy and biomechanics;
- Think about what you are doing;
- Feel it happening from the inside - be aware of your proprioception!

Ideally you want to do lots of little bits of stretching all day long, every day, at every opportunity. Keep yourself as supple as possible all the time.

And do much more of it when you're warming up! Starting gently!

Remember, only you can make it work for you. You are the one doing your stretching. Your instructor will, hopefully, show you how to do it properly but it is up to you to make sure you get it right.

Like any physical skill, stretching takes practice. As you go through the motions, thinking about what you're doing and feeling it from the inside, you will eventually have the experience of feeling it work, of feeling that muscle let go, of feeling those ligaments loosen. That's when you know you're doing it right.

That's when you can start really tuning in to your proprioception and achieve a major breakthrough in exercising for Health, with Fitness following naturally.

Not working on your suppleness:

- Increases your risk of injury;
- Makes you more likely to have aches and pains;
- Reduces the effect of your strength training;
- Reduces the efficiency of your stamina training;
- Makes you get tired more quickly;
- Makes you less and less mobile as you get older.

So the seventh Major Mistake is: **Ignoring the need for suppleness.**

The solution: Proper, safe, self-aware stretching - follow the Golden Guidelines. Remember that stretching is for every day life as well as for sport. Always stretch when warming up. Invest in learning an effective stretching routine for all your most important areas, including learning at least the basics of the relevant anatomy and biomechanics. Learn it from someone who really knows what they are doing and who understands the difference between exercising for Health as opposed to Fitness.

Your best and healthiest exercise:

1   Focuses on health first, fitness second

2   Boosts your physical self-awareness

3   Keeps you at a safe temperature

4   Gives you all the oxygen you need

5   Activates you gradually and safely

6   Safely strengthens you

7   Keeps you supple, loose and mobile

8   ?

9   ?

10   ?

Notes and thoughts:

8
High As a Damaged Kite

"Runner's High" - Have you heard of it?

It's the fantastic feeling people enjoy when they really push themselves in extreme exercise.

They feel happy. They feel great. They feel euphoric. The pain of overworked muscles and injured tissues doesn't bother them.

It's "natural" - so it must be good, right?

It must be safe, right?

Well… actually… no.

Let's think this one through:

Runner's High is caused by a gland in your brain releasing chemicals called endorphins. The endorphin molecules have a very similar shape to the molecules of opiate pain killers - codeine, morphine and heroin.

In fact, that's exactly why opiates work. Their molecules are so similar to endorphins that your brain reacts to them as if they actually were.

That's why the opiates are such powerful pain killers.

And that's why they make you feel so amazing - for a while, until your body gets used to them and starts to need them just to feel normal.

That's what's called "addiction".

Extreme exercise is also addictive. Without a fix of endorphins the addict feels listless, lethargic and generally grumpy. They need their fix just to get back to feeling normal.

Endorphins are only released in response to extreme stress. They are an emergency survival mechanism passed down to you from your remote ancestors.

If you're chasing prey or fleeing from a predator or trying to survive a battle then endorphins definitely have their place. They enable you to keep going when you might give up from pain and exhaustion.

In that context, endorphins are life savers. Your ancestors lived to have children because of them. You wouldn't be here without them!

But they have no place at all in the context of exercising for Health.

Going for the "Runner's High" means you have to push yourself to an extreme - overheating, oxygen debt, dehydration, toxins, shock impacts, muscle strains, exhausted heart, frazzled brain.

Is it really worth it?

How about an alternative?

How about exercising in a way that makes you feel every bit as good as you do with Runner's High but for precisely the opposite reasons?

Runner's High is an illusion, every bit as deceptive as sticking a needle in your arm. And possibly just as dangerous from the harm you do yourself to achieve it. You feel great because your biochemistry is covering up the damage. But it doesn't last and you soon have to damage yourself again to get back to feeling normal.

You know how good you feel after a shower? When you've shampooed your hair and scrubbed yourself down?

You feel refreshed and energised.

Now imagine doing that right the way through your whole body.

Obviously I'm not talking about reaching inside and scrubbing your muscles with soap.

But I am talking about cleansing your system.

I'm talking about exercising so you supply your tissues with all the nutrients they need.

Staying at a safe temperature.

Staying hydrated.

Having plenty of oxygen.

Getting rid of toxins.

Nourishing your muscles, heart and brain.

Treating yourself so well that you have absolutely no need of endorphins at all.

That's a natural high!

At the risk of stating the obvious, the feeling you get from exercising healthily is far, far better than the endorphin rush triggered by harming yourself.

Going for the endorphins:

- Needs you to push yourself to damaging extremes;
- Messes up your biochemistry;
- Stresses your brain;
- Makes you feel terrible when not exercising;
- Makes you biochemically dependent on damaging yourself;
- Risks permanent harm.

So the eighth Major Mistake is: **Thinking Endorphins Are Good.**

The solution: Understand the serious risks involved in pushing yourself into an endorphin high. Exercise so that you nourish and cleanse yourself. Enjoy the physical feeling of healthy fitness. Enjoy the feeling of knowing you are doing yourself good.

Your best and healthiest exercise programme:

1   Focuses on health first, fitness second

2   Boosts your physical self-awareness

3   Keeps you at a safe temperature

4   Gives you all the oxygen you need

5   Activates you gradually and safely

6   Safely strengthens you

7   Keeps you supple, loose and mobile

8   Feels great due to nourishing and cleansing

9   ?

10   ?

9
Rubbish In, Rubbish Out

What happens when you put diesel in a petrol car?

It conks out and stops working, doesn't it? Then you have to drain it and clean it out.

The same principle applies for what you put into yourself.

I've studied biochemistry. I've studied sports science. I've studied nutrition. And yet I too have a history of shoving rubbish in my mouth and still expecting my body to work as if I was giving it high-grade fuel!

I know exactly how easy it is to eat and drink the wrong things, even with all my knowledge and training. It really is no wonder at all that so many people unwittingly make this particular Major Mistake. Mind you, the patient who thought Fruit Pastilles counted as one of their "5 a day" came as a bit of a shock!

Following the right exercise programme, focusing on Health rather than Fitness and avoiding the Major Mistakes, is a huge part of giving you the life you want. It gives you more energy, less stress, less tiredness and fewer aches and pains. It gives you a good, solid, life-long base of robust and happy health from which you can boost your fitness up to peak performance whenever you want.

It's even better and more effective if you combine it with proper eating.

Unless you have a serious eating disorder you can make a significant change just by being more aware of the main food groups and why you need them. Hopefully the brief overview in this chapter will inspire you to learn a bit more on your own too.

Food gives you the molecules that make up your body and the energy that lets it work.

All your energy comes from the sun as light. Plants catch the energy in their leaves and store it in glucose, made from water and carbon dioxide. The glucose releases the energy where it's needed, letting the plant grow - including pulling other nutrients, like nitrogen and minerals, up from the soil and building complex biochemical molecules.

We then eat the plants, or the animals who have already eaten them, and we extract the energy and molecules.

The food you swallow does one of the following:

- Goes straight through and comes out the other end (plus billions of bacteria);
- Gets turned into you;
- Provides energy to keep you alive.

You couldn't live without those bacteria in your gut. They're mostly very friendly. As well as helping you extract maximum nutrition from your food they also protect you from nasty bacteria and other bugs.

You are mainly made of water, from your food as well as from what you drink. You're also made of protein, both structural and biochemical. Even your bones are protein, with lots of minerals added in. Lastly, your body is made up of the molecules used for storing energy - glucose and fat. Plus all that dreaded extra fat that you don't really need!

Some of your food is used for energy straight away. The energy keeps you alive. It keeps you warm, it lets you move, it powers your brain. Above all, the energy helps you maintain the mind-boggling complexity of your body.

Eventually your molecules do fall apart. That's why you keep having to replace them by eating. Your biochemistry then breaks them up and extracts as much energy as possible. The left-over fragments are filtered out of your blood by your kidneys, then kept with water in your bladder until you're ready to empty it. A lot of the carbon becomes carbon dioxide, which is breathed out through your lungs.

OK, so let's have a look at the main food groups…

Fibre: The main reason for your "5 a day". Provides bulk for your gut to get hold of and move food along as it's being digested. Makes it much easier and more comfortable to get rid of when it comes out the other end. Helps clean out your gut, scouring off dead cells and carrying them away - helping your gut work better and getting rid of nasties. Lack of fibre constipates you and can contribute to bowel cancer. Most people don't eat anything like enough fibre. It is extremely likely that you need to eat more than you are doing, or even take supplements. You cannot possibly eat too much of it. The more you eat the better.

Find it in: green leafy vegetables (and their stems); lentils, peas and beans; whole grains; non-starchy root vegetables; fruit. Any of the cabbage family are brilliant - eat loads of broccoli! Meat has no fibre in it at all.

Minerals: The main ones are iron, calcium, sodium and potassium, along with phosphorus and sulphur. You're probably getting plenty of those, possibly too much sodium if you eat a lot of salt or mono-sodium glutamate. Where you might be deficient is in the trace minerals - selenium is an important one, which you can find in nuts. There's also copper, manganese, molybdenum and various others, even gold. They help your biochemistry work properly. You only need tiny amounts but after decades of intensive agriculture they are disappearing from our food. You might benefit from supplements.

Vitamins: Various chemicals essential for your biochemistry. You can't make them yourself so you have to have them in your food. Eating a good variety of different foods should give you enough. Probably no need for supplements unless you have a specific medical condition that stops you absorbing or using them.

Friendly bacteria: Essential for extracting nutrients from food and protecting you against nasties. Find it in live, organic yoghurt. Might be worth supplementing, but the quality of "pro-biotic" supplements varies hugely.

Protein: Great big complex molecules made of thousands of atoms. You're made of protein (and water). All your biochemistry is done by proteins too. There are billions of different proteins, a potentially infinite variety. Your DNA contains the instructions for making yours. All proteins are made from twenty basic building blocks, called amino acids, linked together in long chains then tangled round each other. Protein in your food is broken down then the parts are used for rebuilding your own - a bit like Lego.

There are nine "essential" amino acids, which you have to have in your food. Your biochemistry can make the others for you. No plants have all nine but you can get them all if you eat enough different plants, including different beans, peas and lentils, which also provide fibre. Meat contains all the amino acids. Plus it can have B vitamins that aren't in plants, but it can also be high in fat. Fish is an excellent source of protein.

Carbohydrate: This is your petrol, your fuel, your energy supply. Energy is measured in Calories (kcal) or Kilojoules (kJ).

Simple carbohydrate - sugar (e.g. glucose) - provides energy very quickly, especially if there's lots of oxygen around. Complex carbohydrate - starches - are basically lots of sugar molecules stuck together into long chains. They get chopped up then rebuilt into another form for short-term storage. Or they get chopped up even smaller and rebuilt into fat for long-term storage.

It is very, very likely that you are eating far too much carbohydrate - especially sugar - unless you are burning it off in a manual job or training for an important athletic event.

Any spare carbohydrate is turned into fat. This is probably THE major cause of the obesity crisis. There's a simple formula: Take in more energy than you use up and you put on weight; Use up more energy than you take in and you lose weight.

Huge amounts of sugar are hidden in processed foods - fizzy drinks, fruit juices, biscuits, chocolate, cake, ice cream, sliced white bread, ready-meals - the list is almost endless and they're all best avoided, or at least minimised. Your biochemistry can adjust to expect it and it becomes an addiction. I'm sorry, but that's just the way it is. Alcohol is treated as sugar too! Your choice. Enjoy in moderation! Just be aware of what you are eating and drinking and think twice before doing so.

Cutting out starchy carbohydrates is an easy way to reduce your overall intake. Rice, potatoes, pasta and bread are the main sources you can easily reduce. I stopped having rice with curry years ago - I have lentils instead, which are full of protein and fibre.

Fat: Some fats are good for you and you need them in your diet. Vitamins A, D, E and K are found in the fat in your food. Some of your hormones are made from fats. Your cells would fall apart without fat. The fat under your skin helps keep you warm and it is used for surrounding and protecting your inner organs - although you don't want too much of this "visceral" fat.

Oil from olives, hemp, avocado and a few others are fine. Fish oils - salmon, mackerel, sardine, prawns - are good, although be aware that farmed salmon can be contaminated with pesticides, so it's best to go for wild or organic.

Animal fats are generally not so good although they do no harm in moderation. I would always choose butter over margarine. Synthetic, saturated and "trans" fats should be avoided.

Remember, fat contains much more energy than carbohydrate, which is why your body uses it for long-term energy storage. That's great if there's a serious risk of famine. It's not so good when it's completely unnecessary. It then becomes just a dead weight for you to carry around - putting a strain on your heart, lungs, muscles and joints, making you less agile and mobile and more stressed and tired.

Eating badly:

- Undermines the benefits of your healthy exercise programme;
- Messes up your digestion;
- Confuses your biochemistry;
- Makes you put on weight;
- Strains your body.

So the ninth Major Mistake is: **Eating Badly.**

The solution: Learn about the different food groups. Think about what to eat and what to avoid. Eat more fibre. Eat less carbohydrate, especially sugars. Avoid processed food as much as possible. Eat a varied diet.

Your best and healthiest exercise programme:

1   Focuses on health first, fitness second

2   Boosts your physical self-awareness

3   Keeps you at a safe temperature

4   Gives you all the oxygen you need

5   Activates you gradually and safely

6   Safely strengthens you

7   Keeps you supple, loose and mobile

8   Feels great due to nourishing and cleansing

9   Includes sensible eating

10   ?

10
Too Much, Too Soon

Do I need to say more?

Sorry, there's no way round this one. Too much, too soon, too fast and you're asking for trouble.

No doubt you've seen them advertised, those miraculous diets and exercise programmes that promise to transform you in only a few weeks. Tempting but, face it, they just don't work.

When you look into them they all depend on actively promoting these very Major Mistakes that do so much harm. They are all based on the systems designed for young athletes - high intensity activities that cause burn-out within a few years and significant long-term problems.

Slow, steady, gradual is the only way to get real and permanent results.

Pushing the extremes does you more harm than good. It takes away your health and stops you gaining real fitness.

Striving for quick results puts you straight into the danger zone.

So the tenth Major Mistake is: **Trying for Fast Results**

The solution: Follow an exercise programme that gradually builds. It should lead you, step by step, through a process of learning and self-discovery. You gain lasting health and real fitness.

Your best and healthiest exercise programme:

1   Focuses on health first, fitness second

2   Boosts your physical self-awareness

3   Keeps you at a safe temperature

4   Gives you all the oxygen you need

5   Activates you gradually and safely

6   Safely strengthens you

7   Keeps you supple, loose and mobile

8   Feels great due to nourishing and cleansing

9   Includes sensible eating

10   Gradually leads you to permanent benefits

To Summarise...

The Ten Major Mistakes That Can Make You Unwittingly Fail At Fitness - And Their Solutions

1 Thinking Fitness equals Health - Recognise the difference then focus on Health

2 Lack of physical self-awareness - Tune in to your proprioception

3 Getting hot and sweaty - Have sweat evaporating rather than dripping

4 Getting out of breath - Breathe deep while avoiding panting

5 Not warming up properly - Take more time and do it gradually

6 Exercising with shock impacts and sudden strains - Firm, gradual loading

7 Ignoring the need for suppleness - Follow the Golden Guidelines

8 Thinking endorphins are good - Avoid dangerous extremes

9 Eating badly - Have more fibre and less carbohydrate and eat varied, good quality food

10 Trying for fast results - Gradual progress gets permanent results

Notes and thoughts:

Afterword

As you know, this book is all about how to achieve real and lasting health benefits.

Seeing that instructor getting that stretch so wrong was a turning point for me. How many other instructors were doing the same? Not just for suppleness but for all aspects of health and fitness.

Perhaps I was getting it wrong too. What mistakes was I unwittingly making - doing what I thought was right but getting it wrong without realising?

That's when my strange mixture of training all came together along with my three decades experience helping thousands of people with their health and fitness. I became aware of the fundamental difference between exercising for Health and exercising for Fitness. That's when I fully recognised these 10 Major Mistakes and their extremely important solutions.

As an Osteopath I look at how the whole body works as one whole system and how health problems - pain and illness - occur when that system goes wrong. Then I help the patient's body work better and their health returns. Restoring mobility and suppleness is a major part of treatment. Osteopathy is all about boosting health.

As a Biochemist, Fitness Consultant and Nutritionist, trained in state-of-the-art fitness science, I knew how to get young athletes up to peak performance and how to keep them there as long as possible. I also knew the risks they faced.

As an Advanced Tai Chi Instructor I was aware of the benefits of physical self awareness, of good posture and quality of movement, of correct breathing, of gentle loading of bones, muscles and joints. I had experienced for myself the amazing feeling you get from nourishing and cleansing your tissues - from exercising at a safe temperature and with full oxygenation - and I had been able to compare it with the crazy buzz of endorphins caused by over-exercising.

Having identified these 10 Major Mistakes and realising how much harm they were doing I started looking for existing programmes that took them into account. I was sure I couldn't have been the first person to become aware of them.

But the more I looked the more I had to accept that there was nothing out there. Everything was either far too intense or not intense enough. There was nothing occupying the middle ground and offering a complete system for long-term Health.

So I did it myself!

That's how and why I created Tai-Robics. I took the best of the East and combined it with the best of the West. I've taken the most important parts of Tai Chi and Yoga, simplified them and made them easier and more accessible. I've also taken the best aspects of Western exercise systems, like Aerobics, and removed all the negatives.

The last stage was to put it all together into one, unique system - an exercise programme like no other in that it answers all the 10 Major Mistakes.

Over to you now...! Enjoy!

Visit www.tai-robics.com to register for your local Tai-Robics class, or send an email to help@tai-robics.com for further details

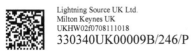